OVERCOMING TENSION

Overcoming Common Problems

OVERCOMING TENSION

Dr Kenneth Hambly
M.B., B.Ch., M.R.C.O.G.

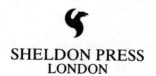

SHELDON PRESS
LONDON

First published in Great Britain in 1983 by
Sheldon Press, SPCK, Marylebone Road, London NW1 4DU

Second Impression 1987

British Library Cataloguing in Publication Data

Hambly, Kenneth
    Overcoming tension.—(Overcoming common problems)
    1. Stress (Psychology)   2. Stress (Physiology)
    3. Stress relaxation
    I. Title   II. Series
    616.8   BF575.S75

    ISBN 0-85969-373-2

Typeset by Memo Typography Ltd
Nicosia, Cyprus
Printed in Great Britain by
Richard Clay Ltd, Bungay, Suffolk

Contents

DEDICATION

To Roger Paxton M. Phil., Ph.D.
a good friend

1

Anxiety States And Phobias: What are They?

There is nothing more shattering for a normal well-adjusted individual than to find that one day quite out of the blue, 'something is wrong'. Perhaps it starts in the cinema or theatre, or in a crowded shop. It might be at home with friends. There might be a feeling of unease, perhaps of dizziness. There might be a speeding up of the heart and a general feeling of panic. It has happened to many people.

It happened to a friend of mine. He is a young professional man with a wife and family. He was apparently happy, well-adjusted and at ease with himself. One night he was at the cinema when he began to feel unwell. He felt dizzy and tearful and had to leave the cinema. The feeling left him quickly, but the experience disturbed him.

During the ensuing weeks he began to have bouts of diarrhoea and severe headaches. He also began to feel unsteady on his feet, particularly in the restaurant where he went for lunch. He began to take lunch in the office and stopped going out with his wife in the evenings. He had developed an anxiety state.

This is the way an anxiety state begins for many people. Sometimes it starts more slowly with occasional feelings of tightness in the chest, or occasional headaches. There may be a tremor, or a feeling of tearfulness in company. This may be the way it happened to you. You may have had no idea what was wrong with you, or more likely you may have had a good idea that it was something to do with your 'nerves'.

What is an anxiety state?

One way or another, you have developed an anxiety state. So what is it and what is a phobia? Why do they occur? Anxiety itself is easy to understand. It is part of everyone's life. Anyone who has sat an examination, been to an interview, taken a driving test or made a speech knows all about anxiety. There is that feeling of apprehension. There may be a tremor or the nervous interviewee may get diarrhoea. No one would consider that unusual. Everyone, or almost everyone, suffers in the same way. Anxiety is a normal response to a stressful situation. It is a physical response to stress, and in a way it is a hangover from our distant past. If prehistoric man was chased by a wild animal his body produced a chemical substance called adrenalin, which is released into the bloodstream from two little glands situated above the kidneys. The stimulation for this release comes from the nervous system. It helped him by instantly 'tuning up' his entire body, giving him the strength and speed to escape. The effect of adrenalin is mostly on the muscles.

The same thing happens today if you are chased by a bull. You develop a strength and speed you didn't know you had. Nowadays however, the stresses are often more subtle. A tough interview is a reasonable substitute for a charging bull, but the physical response is the same. It is a normal reaction.

If you experience this sort of reaction without there being any obvious or immediate stress, or in response to a situation which other people might not find stressful, then you are suffering from what is termed an *anxiety state*. It is exactly the same physical reaction which you might experience before an examination, but now there is no examination, no interview, no obvious external stress. The anxiety is normal, but it is happening in abnormal circumstances.

What is a phobia?

A phobia is simply the occurrence of the symptoms of anxiety in a

2

particular situation which most people wouldn't find stressful. The symptoms might occur in a shop, a cinema, a crowded church or on an aircraft. Some people get symptoms in a lift, or when confronted by a dog or cat. You can be phobic about anything, and that includes the harmless spider. Almost everyone has a phobia and in general the public understands and accepts them. The image of the housewife standing on a chair to escape from the harmless mouse is well known. No one thinks it odd.

A person with a phobia gets his symptoms in response to a particular stress. The person with an anxiety state gets his symptoms more often, perhaps most of the time. Often, however, the anxious person's symptoms are worse in specific situations. They may be worse if he has to go shopping, or travel on a bus. Likewise, the person with a phobia tends to be anxious at other times. The two conditions are closely inter-related.

What causes anxiety states and phobias?

If you suffer from an anxiety state you are entitled to wonder why? Why should you go from being a perfectly capable competent individual to being someone who physically shakes at the thought of going out to a party. What has caused your anxiety state?

The answer is not easy to find, and there are conflicting views. Perhaps no one knows the whole answer. We are all different individuals and we have different personalities. Some are brash and extrovert, some are quiet and shy. Some tend to be more anxious than others. We inherit these tendencies from our parents.

Learning responses

It is also true that we are constantly learning throughout our lives. Not only do we learn things consciously, but our body also learns without our being aware of the fact. As an infant our

3

bladder learns to control itself, which saves us the embarrassment of spending our entire lives in nappies. We learn to balance and to walk. We learn to respond to danger, and to distinguish what is dangerous. Our bodies learn when to produce adrenalin and when not to.

It is thought that in some individuals, this learning process goes wrong. Our bodies learn to produce adrenalin too easily and we thus become prone to developing an anxiety state.

If you are involved in a car accident you may become anxious at the prospect of travelling in a car again. You may tremble and feel sick when you are in a car or at the thought of going in a car. Your body has learned to produce adrenalin at the prospect of travelling in a car. You may become fearful of travelling in cars and actually *avoid* travelling in cars. If you avoid difficult situations there is no way that you can 'unlearn' the physical reaction that your body has erroneously learnt. You have developed a car phobia. You are more likely to do this if you have an inherited tendency to be anxious.

This is a rather crude example of how an anxiety state or phobia may start. Very few of us are involved in car accidents. Most anxiety states develop much more slowly, usually over a period of years, and sometimes from early childhood. We react to situations throughout our lives, and we unconsciously learn what our responses should be. Some of us simply learn the wrong responses.

Pavlov's dogs

There is a famous experiment conducted by Pavlov in which some dogs were fed at the same time as a bell was rung. The dogs learned to associate the ringing of the bell with the production of food. The dogs, like all good dogs, would salivate when the food was produced. Soon they would salivate when the bell was rung, confident that food would soon follow. They associated the ringing of the bell with food. Eventually they would salivate when the bell was rung whether the food was produced or not. They would

4

salivate whether they wanted to or not. Their bodies had learned to respond to the *idea* of food.

You can see that it is quite possible to develop unpleasant symptoms when presented with an abstract concept. In the analogy of the individual who developed the car phobia, his body had learned to respond to the idea of travelling in the car. It is not unusual for someone to produce adrenalin and experience symptoms in anticipation of an event. Often the anticipation is worse than the event itself.

These abnormal responses are learned in small ways throughout life, starting in early childhood. We learn all sorts of things, and most of our learning is beneficial. Bad or inappropriate responses can also be learned. There is hope however. Things which are learned can also be unlearned, and it is this simple truth which offers us the possibility for treatment. Our inappropriate responses can be unlearned and more suitable responses substituted.

Sigmund Freud

Not everyone agrees with this concept. Freud thought that psychological states were produced by subconscious conflicts. You will undoubtedly have seen films where someone lies on the analyst's couch and tries to unravel these supposed conflicts. I am not at all convinced by this theory. No one has ever shown that such conflicts have produced anxiety states.

I feel that it is wrong to dwell on the possible subconscious causes of your anxiety state. Just accept that you have a problem and set about treating it. Accept that you have developed responses which have been wrongly learned and set about the business of learning the correct ones. It sounds easy but in fact it requires a lot of attention and application. This book will tell you how to go about it.

Meet Mrs Jean F.

I want to introduce you to some people who have had anxiety states and who have learned to control them, overcome them and to live normal lives. I do not pretend that they never get any symptoms. They do get occasional problems, but they control them and are not excessively bothered by them. They have no fear. They lead happy lives. The first is Mrs Jean F. I will tell you about her because it will give you some idea what can be done and how it can be done.

Jean was thirty-four years of age and had always been healthy. She had never had any psychiatric or 'nervous' troubles. Her friends thought of her as a normal outgoing young woman. She did not go out to work, but looked after her husband and two young sons on a new housing estate. She had been a little unwell for a few weeks and had thought of consulting her doctor, but she had been reluctant to do so because she really could not put her finger on what was wrong.

One morning she felt a little worse. She decided to go shopping anyway and set off for the shops. She went first to the supermarket. She felt apprehensive about going in, but there seemed to be no reason not to. She went in but after a few minutes began to feel very unwell indeed. She began to sweat. Her pulse pounded and she began to tremble. Not unnaturally she rushed from the shop. She managed to return home and immediately called her general practitioner who came within an hour. By the time he arrived, her symptoms had settled and she was more or less back to normal.

Her G.P. examined her thoroughly and came back to see her the next day, when he took blood tests. Again he could find no physical problems and reassured her. Jean continued to feel unwell. She did not feel like going out, but the next day she went shopping to the supermarket again with the same result. She was again seen by her G.P., but this time he discussed her problems with her. He diagnosed her as having an anxiety state and ex-

6

plained it to her. He told her that she had become phobic about going out and particularly about going into shops.

He outlined a system of treatment which involved learning relaxation exercises and practising deep relaxation. He persuaded her to keep a diary of her symptoms in an effort to define those symptoms accurately and the exact situations which brought them on. He saw her again in a week.

By this time she was feeling better, although she had not felt able to go out. She was managing to relax well and this was helping her. Her doctor urged her to begin to go out again. She arranged to go to the corner shop accompanied by a friend who she told about her problem. She went every day and made one purchase only. She kept going until she felt confident enough to go by herself. She had panic attacks but could manage them, and she found that she did not have to leave the shop.

Her confidence returned enough for her to go to the local post office, which was not far away. She did this for a week, and gradually extended her activity, being advised by her doctor. She was feeling better and better, and soon was able to resume normal activity, despite occasional problems with symptoms. Life, which was for a time difficult and distressing, is again happy and fulfilling.

2

Your Symptoms: What Causes Them?

You may be suffering from a condition which you find confusing and frightening. It probably affects your entire life. It alters the way you behave in public and limits the things you can do. You will hate it, and may hate yourself for having it. Can it really be reduced to a list of physical symptoms?

No it can't. An anxiety state is a complex condition, and people react to it in different ways. Behind every anxiety state however there *is* a list of symptoms. If we are to begin to tackle our anxiety state, this is a good place to start. Physical symptoms are tangible. They are not frightening. If you can identify your own physical symptoms then your entire anxiety state will become less frightening, and as a result, much easier to come to terms with.

The next time you feel unwell, sit down in a quiet corner and have a good look at yourself. Try to relax your muscles. The exercises later in this book will help you to do this. Relax your muscles. Now try to see just what is wrong. Are your muscles tense? Are they sore, perhaps in your neck or legs? Is this making you feel dizzy? Are you sweating? Is your stomach upset?

Try to list the things you physically feel. It may help you if you write them down. As soon as you have established just why you feel the way you do, you will be less disturbed and more relaxed. The known is always less frightening than the unknown.

These symptoms you are experiencing are normal adrenalin responses which you are experiencing in an extreme form at a time when other people might not experience them. To help you investigate your symptoms I have made a list of the more common ones. Remember that no one suffers from all of them. You may recognize one or two.

Muscle tension

This is certainly the most common symptom. You may feel tension in the muscles of the jaw, neck, back, and sometimes chest or legs. You may wake up with sore teeth from teeth clenching all night. There may be nail marks on the palms of your hands. You certainly will not have slept in a restful way, and you wake up tired. You will be tense during the day as well. You tension can persist for hours. It will be felt in the muscles of your face, so that your whole face feels tight and sore. Your face is a mask and smiling seems impossible. If you smile you feel that your face may crack. These symptoms are so common that almost anyone with an anxiety state can describe them.

Headaches

Tension headaches, which everyone experiences from time to time, are caused by a tightening up of the muscles in the back of the neck. Your neck stiffens up and your scalp becomes tight, so that there is a feeling of pressure on the scalp. The pain is often felt behind the eyes. People with tension states are particularly prone to this type of headache. If you think that you have a tension headache try pressing on the muscles in the back of your neck with your thumbs. You will find that these muscles are sore to the touch. Massage will sometimes help these muscles to relax. So will relaxation exercises. Persistent headaches should be investigated by your doctor. If no cause can be found, you may have to deal with them yourself using techniques described in this book.

Pains

You may feel pain in your shoulder or chest, or perhaps in your legs. Of course pains can be caused by many things, and if you have pain you must be sure that there is no physical cause for it. This will necessitate a visit to your doctor. If no physical cause can be found for your pain, it might be that your pain is caused by the contraction of groups of muscles. Excessive production of adrenalin not only makes all of your muscles contract, it can also make groups of muscles go into spasm. Muscles in spasm can be very painful, as anyone who has had a pulled muscle will know. If you have severe chest pain, it may be muscular in origin. In that way it is caused directly by your anxiety state. Your severe chest pain may not be caused by your heart. It may be cramping, sore muscles in your chest wall.

Excessive fatigue

Many people consult their doctors because they feel tired all the time. It is a common sensation which you may well have experienced. You may have gone to your doctor, been examined and investigated and nothing abnormal found. It might just be that you feel tired because you *are* tired. You may have been sleeping all night, but you may not have been sleeping in a restful way. If you wake up with a sore jaw from clenching your teeth all night then you can hardly be well rested. Your muscles may remain tense all day. You can hardly be surprised if you begin to feel tired. How could you feel anything else?

Tremor

You may be one of the people who has a hand tremor. It may be worse if someone is looking at you or if you have to perform an intricate task. A tremor is a common problem. Many people who do not have anxiety states suffer from a mild tremor of their hands. It only becomes a problem if it intrudes into your life. For a few people it is a dominant symptom and a problem. It is very embarrassing not to be able to carry a cup and saucer. A tremor is caused by an increase in muscle tension.

Dizziness

Dizziness is one of the most disturbing symptoms which someone suffering from an anxiety state can experience. It is also one of the most common. It can make you feel insecure. It is associated with a feeling of disorientation and you may think that you are going to pass out. You may just feel that you are not yourself. You feel different. If your doctor can find no physical cause for this sensation, what is going on?

I am quite sure that the cause of this bizarre symptom is an imbalance in the tension in the muscles of the neck. One of these muscles goes into spasm, or the muscles on one side of the neck contract more than the muscles on the other. Every muscle and joint in the body has receptors which tell our brain what that muscle or joint is doing. These receptors are particularly important in the neck, where they give the brain information which helps with our balance mechanism. If you get severe contractions on one side and not the other then you feel odd, insecure and dizzy. You can test this theory by pressing on the muscles in your neck when you feel this way. If you push your thumbs into the muscles at the back of the neck you will find that the muscles on one side only are in spasm. The muscles will be tight and if you press hard you will feel pain on that side of your head and sometimes into your eye or jaw.

Doing this can also make you feel a little sick. No wonder you feel a little peculiar. It is a sensation only. Tension in neck muscles will never make you fall. Try a little massage. Take a few aspirin. Do not be frightened by this sensation. That feeling that you are falling to the side is just another sensation produced by muscle spasm. Accept it for what it is. Either relax it away or try to ignore it. It is the fear of the symptom which causes you the problems, not the symptom itself.

Palpitations

People with anxiety states occasionally feel that their heart is

11

beating quickly, or that their heart is missing a beat. Your doctor may tell you that you are having palpitations. What is really happening is that the heart has a quick extra beat, and this is followed by a pause which you may notice and find unpleasant. The phenomenon is caused by the direct action of adrenalin on the heart. Your heart has special receptors which respond to adrenalin, and if you produce too much adrenalin your heart will react. Palpitations can be frequent and can last for some time. Palpitations can do you no harm. They are an annoyance, but there is nothing wrong with your heart.

Diarrhoea

Some people complain of a phenomenon which is not so much diarrhoea as loose stools. It may be worse in the morning or before a stressful event. We are all familiar with the problem before interviews and the like. We have had butterflies in the tummy and had to go to the lavatory. Again this is the direct action of adrenalin on the receptors in the gut, which speeds up and produces diarrhoea. You may experience it on occasions when other people might not expect to experience it. It's the same old story.

Stomach upsets

I once heard a television personality describe how guests on his show, many of them experienced performers, were physically sick in their dressing rooms before appearing before the cameras. This is a straight stress reaction which is not confined to television personalities. Your stomach produces too much acid. The muscles in your stomach wall tighten up giving you extreme indigestion. You feel ill and you may even vomit. It is only your body overreacting.

Difficulty getting your breath

Sometimes you may feel that you have difficulty completely filling your lungs. You breathe deeply but cannot seem to get a satisfactory breath. If your doctor listens to your chest there is nothing out of the ordinary to hear. A chest X-ray is normal. It is a subjective sensation which you experience.

I am not too sure how this one works, but the phenomenon of increased muscle tension is so common that it surely contributes to this feeling. I think that the muscles between the ribs become tight and as a result there is a feeling of constriction. It is an annoying feeling but it can do you no harm. It is usually not constant, but comes on at times of stress, such as entering a room full of strangers.

Difficulty swallowing

This is another problem which is worse in a stressful situation. You feel you have to keep swallowing o clear the saliva from your mouth. You feel as if you are going to choke. It is caused by a tightening of the muscles in your gullet. You can create a similar, though not identical, sensation by pushing your tongue into the roof of your mouth. When you are stressed, you start to swallow, and once you have started you do not seem to be able to stop. It is sometimes associated with an 'indigestion' feeling. It is that sick feeling which makes you keep swallowing. If you just stay where you are and try to relax it will pass off.

Sometimes you will get the feeling when you are eating a meal, usually in company. This time the gullet itself tightens up to the extent that the food will just not go down. If you sit and relax, breathing slowly, the contraction will disappear and the food will at last go down. Check with your doctor, and if there is nothing physically wrong with you, it is again a matter of learning the right responses.

13

Tearfulness

There are two types of tearfulness. One is associated with depression. You cry because you feel sad. If you feel depressed then you should see your doctor who will be able to help you.

The other kind of tearfulness is quite different. It is more a feeling of impending tears than tears of real sadness. You feel as if you are on the verge of breaking down and crying. You usually don't actually cry, but the fear of crying is just as bad and just as socially debilitating. The sensation occurs when the muscles of the face are tight and contracted. Tears are almost squeezed out by tension in the muscles around the eyes. Your face is held like a mask, and you feel that if you drop your guard for a second you will break down and cry. It is a distressing symptom which makes meeting and talking with other people difficult. It is most unlikely that you ever will cry in these circumstances. There is no reason why you should. It is simply that you are physically tense. The fear of what might happen is worse than the sensation itself.

Bladder problems

Occasionally men have problems with their bladder. They may have a sensation that they should pass more water after they have actually finished. They may dribble a little after passing water. There can be physical reasons for these problems, particularly in older men. If no physical cause can be found, then it may just be contraction of the muscles of the neck of the bladder. These muscles contract, trapping a little water in the tube from the bladder and giving a most unpleasant sensation. The sensation can be relieved by pressing on the tube from the bladder as it passes under the pubic bones, just behind the scrotum. It is like scratching an itch. You can 'milk' the last few drops of urine from the tube. It is a trick which can give immense relief.

Panic attacks

Panic attacks are the most disturbing of the phenomena which the person who has an anxiety state can experience. In such an attack powerful symptoms come on suddenly, usually in a public place such as a supermarket.There is an increase in the heart rate. You feel dizzy and sweat. You may shake or be short of breath. This is an emergency. You have to get out. You are terrified, and no wonder. Symptoms like these would terrify anybody.

A panic attack is no more and no less than the sudden onset of a set of symptoms. They come over you in a wave. You feel that you have to leave the building before you collapse or even die. If only you could stand still and even relax for a minute. These attacks are quickly over. If you can have the courage to wait for those few seconds you will find that the attack reaches a climax very quickly and then slowly passes off. After the attack you feel as right as rain. You will also find that no one has noticed that anything is wrong.

After your panic attack it is worth wondering why it happened in that place and at that time. Was it because you were sweating due to excessive heat? Was your stomach upset? Often your body misinterprets perfectly normal symptoms as being caused by anxiety instead of by the simple physical cause. So when you get that tingling feeling down your back when you start to sweat, your body decides that this is the cue for the release of adrenalin and you have a panic attack.

It is often fear of a panic attack which keeps agoraphobics indoors, and other people out of shops, buses and planes. It is easy to learn to deal with a panic attack. More about that later.

Fear of the symptoms

That is the end of my symptom list. You may be able to think of others and perhaps make a list of your own. But can you reduce this fearful, terrifying, anxiety state to a list of physical symptoms? I am sure that you can. Basically that is what it is. An anxiety state is a collection of symptoms produced by an over-active nervous system. Of course there are other things you could say about it. Someone who is unable to leave the house because of a phobic fear of the outside might be very offended if he was told that his problem could be reduced to a list of symptoms. Yet such a person does not have a fear of the outside. Certainly not. That would be irrational. He does, however, have a profound fear of the symptoms which he gets if he does venture outside, and that is very understandable. I am sure that someone who has not experienced the symptoms produced by an anxiety state could never believe the intensity of those symptoms. He would not believe the fear which they produce.

It is the fear of the symptoms which is disabling, not the symptoms themselves. There is good evidence to show that people who suffer from anxiety states are as physically healthy as anyone else in the community. They live as long as anyone else. Your symptoms can do you no harm. Your anxiety state or phobia cannot damage your body.

If your symptoms can do you no harm, why are you so scared of them? It is time you came to terms with your anxiety state and stopped letting it rule your life.

3

How Can Your Mind
Produce Physical Symptoms?

I think it is worth spending a little time considering the way your body works. Many people who say their nerves are bad have no idea what they really mean. It is much easier to deal with your problems if you understand exactly what is going on, so I will deal briefly with the workings of the nervous system. It is a bit more complicated than you may think.

Everyone understands that they have nerves which transmit and receive messages. If you touch something cold, your brain receives the message from your finger and you are aware that the object is cold. Similarly if you want to move your arm, a message goes from your brain to your arm and the arm moves. This is only a very small part of the story. The fact is that everything which happens in the body is under the control of your nervous system, but you are only aware of a very small part of what is happening.

Take the simple business of standing. Nothing much to that? There is more to it than there seems to be. Your muscles have a certain tension in them. If that tension wasn't there you would collapse in a heap like a puppet with its strings cut. Messages go from the muscles to indicate the weight which the individual muscles are bearing, and messages go back to the muscles to maintain or alter the tension necessary to bear that weight. It is a constantly changing pattern of messages which you are not aware of. The system is automatic. If it goes out of balance you could get too much tension. Eventually you would become aware of it. It would be uncomfortable. It could cause pain or a tremor.

There are many other functions of the nervous system of which we are not aware. What makes our pupils dilate or contract, for example? What regulates the heart? What closes off the blood vessels of our skin when we are cold? What makes the muscles of the bowel work more quickly to give us diarrhoea?

All of these functions are controlled by the automatic part of the nervous system. It is properly called the *autonomic* nervous system and without it we could do nothing. Normally it behaves itself very well and we are just not aware of its actions. In times of stress we become all too aware of its workings, and people with anxiety states may be aware of its actions all the time.

The autonomic nervous system doesn't only work through the nerves in the body. It is even more clever than that. It can work by causing special glands to secrete chemicals into the bloodstream. These chemicals have actions which are similar to those produced by nervous impulses, except that their effects are felt over the entire body and not in one isolated part.

The most important of these chemicals is adrenalin. It is the body's immediate answer to stress. It prepares the whole body for action. In the right situation its release is vital. If it is released in the wrong or inappropriate situation, it can have uncomfortable effects.

Here are some of the actions of adrenalin on different organs. You may be only too familiar with some of them.

Heart: Adrenalin makes the heart beat faster and more strongly.

Blood vessels: Arteries have muscles in their walls. This controls the amount of blood flowing through them. Adrenalin makes the arteries in the skin contract, directing the blood to other more important places, such as muscles.

Eyes: The muscles in the eye relax and the pupils dilate to facilitate 'far' vision.

Muscles: Adrenalin makes all the big muscles in the body become tense.

The digestive system: The bowel is lined by a muscle coat. The muscles in this lining contract in sequence, pushing the contents

18

of the gut through. Adrenalin makes these muscles contract more quickly, speeding up the transport of the bowel contents and in this way causing diarrhoea.

The lungs: The bronchioles, those tubes which carry air into the lungs, have a muscular lining. They dilate to allow more air to enter. The rate at which we breathe speeds up as well.

The pancreas: Insulin production is speeded up. It makes sugars available to the muscles to fuel sudden action.

Sweat glands: Adrenalin makes your sweat glands operate.

You can see that one hormone has many effects. All of them are essential if you are in danger. It means that you can act quickly. What happens though if the adrenalin is produced in just a small excess all of the time? Or if it is produced in large amounts at inappropriate times? You can work out from the list of the actions of adrenalin just what the effects might be, and how the individual might feel.

Adrenalin does not act uniformly. It can cause some of its effects without others. This is because the organs have different receptors which make them respond in particular ways to the secretion of adrenalin. In some ways, not as yet well understood, adrenalin can cause one muscle to contract more than another. This is why we can get a contraction of the muscles of one side of the neck only. Muscles in contraction cause pain, in this case a headache.

It is not important to remember all these details about the way your body works. It is certainly not essential for treatment, but if you understand what is happening to your body you may begin to appreciate why treatment is so difficult. If your anxiety state can be reduced to a group of physical symptoms brought on by the secretion of adrenalin, why can't it be cured by taking a pill? It's a good question, but unfortunately there is no pill which will stop the action of adrenalin.

To understand why, you must remember that an anxiety state is a mixture of a physical and a psychological state. The adrenal

19

glands are under the direct control of the nervous system. In fact they are part of the nervous system. We are talking about an imbalance rather than a disease. It is a subtle condition which is difficult to treat medically.

It could be compared to the disease, thyrotoxicosis, which is a condition in which the thyroid gland overacts. It produces effects very similar to an anxiety state, and it can be difficult for doctors to differentiate between the two conditions. The thyroid gland controls the body's metabolism. If you produce too much of the thyroid hormone you will have a tremor and you may sweat. Thyrotoxicosis is an entirely physical disease well understood by doctors. An overactive thyroid gland can be controlled by drugs, or sometimes by surgery. When the condition is treated the patient returns to normal.

There is no known medication which will control the secretions of the adrenal gland. The glands themselves are tiny and not amenable to surgery. Adrenalin is essential to life, but it is produced in tiny quantities, almost too small to measure. It is a very potent substance indeed.

In an anxiety state there is nothing wrong with the adrenal gland. The problem is with the way the entire nervous system reacts. Again, there is nothing fundamentally wrong with the nervous system. The basic fault is a psychological one. It is your psyche which has taught your nervous system to over-react. There is no point in starting to treat the adrenal gland. It is only doing its job. Likewise the nervous system is only doing what it has learnt to do. Effective treatment must start with our minds.

What we have is a psychological state with physical manifestations. We must treat the whole thing together. There is no other way to proceed.

4

How Can We Learn to Face Difficult Situations?

I am willing to bet that there are some situations which you find difficult to face. When you are in that situation your symptoms are worse. It may be so bad that you avoid those situations altogether. Perhaps it is just that in those situations your symptoms are a little worse than usual.

There are some situations which would be difficult for anyone to face. Walking on to the stage of the National Theatre and delivering a soliloquy from *Hamlet* would be difficult for anyone. What has happened to you is that your threshold for difficult situations has been lowered. You may now get your symptoms when you go into a supermarket. The symptoms experienced are exactly the same as those experienced by the actor at the National Theatre, but you are getting them in the supermarket. You must learn to overcome your symptoms in exactly the same way as the actor. You must practise and rehearse.

Let us consider how one lady did this. Do you remember Mrs Jean F., the lady I introduced earlier? She was experiencing excessive sweating, a tremor and a rapid pounding pulse when she entered some local shops. This became worse until she couldn't go out at all without getting her symptoms. Her friends did her shopping for her, so that she was able to avoid the situations she found difficult.

If Jean was to continue to avoid going out, or at least to avoid going into shops, she could never learn to control her symptoms in those stressful situations. Worse than that, she might stop going out altogether and become housebound. This is the way agoraphobia starts. It is tragic because it is unnecessary.

The first steps

The first thing that Jean did was to learn relaxation exercises. She was able to do this in the quiet of her own home. When she had learned how to achieve relaxation she began to imagine herself going out to the shops, perhaps just to the corner shop. She did this whilst she was relaxing. She had a good imagination and she found that she could recreate the symptoms she experienced whilst shopping during a relaxation session. She was thus able to practise controlling her symptoms in her own home using relaxation exercises. She could simply relax them away.

As soon as she could, Jean began to go out. She did not rush to the busy supermarket, she began with a short walk quite close to the house. She went with friends, and when she was confident doing this, and only then, she started going into shops.

She worked to a plan. Initially she went to the corner shop with a friend and made one purchase. She kept doing this for a week until she was quite confident in that situation. She went at a busy time and stayed for a while. She had occasional panic attacks, and other less alarming symptoms, but she managed to stay in the shop and ride out the attacks. The more often she did this, the more confident she became. As confidence returned she was able to progress to more stressful situations. She worked to a plan she had written out at the beginning of treatment.

Setbacks

Jean had setbacks. It wasn't all plain sailing. On occasions she had to leave a shop or return home before she planned to. On those occasions she simply went back to a less stressful situation and proceeded as before. Within five weeks she was shopping in the supermarket. She was not completely comfortable. She continued to have her symptoms and she did have an occasional panic attack, but her symptoms no longer alarmed her and she was confident about her future.

For Jean's treatment to be successful she had to understand its

22

aims and be prepared to do a lot of work. She had to have the courage to experience her symptoms in public before overcoming her problems. If she hadn't been prepared to do this, there is every chance she would have become housebound.

I have used Jean's case to illustrate the method of treatment. Hers is a very common presentation of the problem. Many, many people have trouble going into crowded places. Often queueing at the checkout is the problem. People can get symptoms anywhere where they feel trapped. It might be a bus or a plane, or perhaps just a room full of people.

For some people, and they are very much in the minority, there seems to be constant anxiety without a phobic element. The principles of treatment are the same, except that perhaps there is more emphasis on relaxation. It is likely however, that there is a phobic element to these anxiety states if it is looked for hard enough.

Principles of treatment

The same treatment methods can be applied to any problem. It takes a little ingenuity to adapt them, but it can always be done. Working out your treatment programme can be interesting. Putting it into practice can be challenging, but it does produce results and so it is rewarding. It can also be enjoyable.

The stages of treatment can be summarized as follows:

1   Make sure you understand the principles of treatment. Be prepared to read the relevant chapters of this book a few times.

2   Make a list of the symptoms you get. That isn't as easy as it sounds. You may not be aware that you are getting specific symptoms. You may just feel unwell. When you are next feeling bad, note exactly what physical problems you are experiencing. It could be anything from stomach churning to tension in the neck muscles. These are the things you are setting out to improve.

3   Keep a diary of the symptoms you experience and of the

23

situations which make them worse.

4   When you have been doing this for a while, write down your least threatening situation. That is the one which only just brings on your symptoms in a very minor way.

5   Write down your most feared situation.

6   List 4 or 5 'in between' situations in order of increasing difficulty. These should all be situations which you can practise easily. Use your local knowledge to make out a realistic programme.

7   While you are doing this, learn to relax at home. Practise behaving in a relaxed way in public. Sit and move in a relaxed way.

8   Start practising your easiest situation. If you can't do it in reality, do it in your mind at home. Practise at least once every day. Only progress when you are comfortable and confident in that situation.

9   Progress in slow stages. It will take weeks.

10   Stick to your plan. Don't be tempted to hurry things. Don't test yourself by trying things that are not in the plan and may be too difficult for you.

You can see how this system was applied by the lady who had her symptoms in shops. She had no difficulty finding situations to practise because there are plenty of shops. What about someone who gets symptoms in a thunderstorm or in a strong wind? It isn't easy to practise facing a thunderstorm every day. It may be that your symptoms are produced by very subtle things, such as the presence of a particularly aggressive individual. How can you arrange that?

Rehearsal and practice

It isn't always easy to 'set up' situations which you can practise. It may require a lot of ingenuity and imagination, particularly the latter. You can always practise things in your imagination. It isn't as good as doing it in real life, but if that is all that is possible, then it is better than nothing by far. Your diary may help you to pinpoint other similar areas which you can practise. If your stresses are subtle, then you will have to think up situations which you will be able to practise every day.

James M

It is often easier to think about real people with real problems. The problems are not always straightforward. James M. is a young man who had a responsible job as manager of a local branch of a chain store. He was usually fit and was not aware of any particular problems with tension. He was in the throes of a divorce action, but seemed to be taking it in his stride.

One day whilst walking in the city he developed severe pain in his chest. He was able to walk to the nearest hospital where he had various tests. He was kept for observation overnight, but allowed home in the morning when all the investigations were found to be negative.

He had another attack at home. Again his pain was severe and he was admitted. Nothing was found to be wrong. On careful questioning it was thought that he might be suffering from an anxiety state, and that his pain might be due to tension in his chest muscles. James was quite unable to accept this explanation, but he agreed to keep a careful diary of his symptoms and what he was doing when they came on. He was told that when his pain came on he was to sit quietly and wait for it to ease.

In the next week he did get the pain again. It occurred after an argument with a customer. He sat down and rested but it did not go away and he had to go home. He felt that he could not face work in case the pain came on. He was frightened of what might happen.

His diary revealed that he was having other symptoms. He had a tremor at work which was worse when there was some stress.

25

He also felt tension in his neck and face muscles which was worse in company.

He was persuaded to practise relaxation exercises and to go out to his local pub as he had been doing before his pain started. Whenever his pain came on he would go straight home. He could not be persuaded to stay where he was and let the pain pass off. He did not have that confidence.

He found that he could manage and even practise his other symptoms in company, but he could not manage the pain.

It was necessary to prove to James that his pain really could not do him any harm. With a little persuasion he agreed to do some exercises when his pain came on. He did press-ups, and to his surprise the pain did not get worse, and even more surprising, nothing terrible happened to him. His confidence grew. He practised difficult situations at home whilst doing his relaxation exercises. In particular he imagined facing aggressive customers. His pulse rate would rise and he would feel tense, but he could control the worst of his symptoms with relaxation techniques.

James returned to work again quite soon. He stayed out of the shop at first, but gradually took more interest in the customers and was eventually able to seek out difficult individuals and deal with them. When he got his pain, he would simply sit down for a few minutes.

In that same year he won an award from his firm for having the highest turnover in the country for a branch of his size.

It is not always easy to find the correct approach to your problem. It may require a little study. It will certainly require a lot of effort and courage, but it can be done. Many people have done it before you.

5

Other Situations Which Can Produce Tension

This chapter should not be considered in isolation. All that has been said about relaxation and rehearsal is just as important in the situations described here as with the other examples which have been given. You should still learn to relax and you should still sit down with a pencil and paper and work out your approach. The following is not a comprehensive list. It is merely a list of some of the more common situations which people find difficult, with some suggestions on how you should deal with them.

Lifts

If you get your symptoms in lifts you have to start practising in lifts. Chose the one which is least threatening, and which you can use often. Chose a time when there are likely to be no other travellers, particularly if your problem seems to be related to the close proximity of others. Prepare yourself well for the first journey in the way already described. Take a friend if you can. Then call your chosen lift and get in. Breathe slowly and relax. Press the button for the next floor. When the door closes continue to relax. When you get to the next floor get out and congratulate yourself on doing something pretty courageous. Repeat the procedure as often as you can. Come back as often as you can and practise until you are confident. Then start to go up two floors. Progress in a planned way, with situations of increasing difficulty. Do not test yourself. Progress until you can manage to ride to the top floor in a lift full of people.

Buses and trains

Many people have severe symptoms when they travel on public transport. Finding buses and perhaps trains to practise on is easy enough, particularly if you live in a city. Remember that you must practise every day, so choose a bus route where you can do this. Plan your campaign carefully. Go and watch the bus you intend to travel on. Watch it stop. Watch the passengers getting on. Go home and go through your journey in your imagination, relaxing whilst you do it.

When it comes to making your first bus journey set yourself a target. One bus stop might be enough. If you have someone who will help you, take them along. Choose a quiet time, when there are not too many people waiting. Stand quietly at the bus stop breathing slowly and deeply. Let any feelings of panic flow over you. When the bus comes, get in and sit by the door.

While the bus is moving, sit comfortably, breathe slowly, and when your stop comes get off slowly and quietly. Practise often and make your journeys longer. Choose a more busy time and be prepared to ride out any panic attacks which might occur.

If you get your symptoms in trains there is a greater problem. If you are not a commuter you will not have much access to trains. Travelling on an inter-city train is rather like travelling on an aircraft, and the section about planes deals with this sort of problem. When you get on, you can't very easily get off. If possible you should practise on a local train.

All the remarks made about buses apply to practise on trains. Plan your first outing well. Go to the station and watch the trains until you are confident that you can travel up the line to the next station. Take along a friend and organize your transport back (if there isn't a suitable train). Go to the station early. Relax while you wait for the train. When it comes, get on quietly and sit by the door. You will certainly feel apprehensive, but the anticipation is usually worse. When you finally do it, it isn't as bad as you thought it would be. Your nervous system will react, but it can do

28

you no harm. In a way it is interesting feeling it react so long as you know what is going on. When you reach the next station you will feel exhilarated by your achievement.

Cars

People get symptoms in cars for all types of different reasons. It isn't usually the car itself which brings on symptoms. It is something outside the car, or some aspect of driving. If you are a passenger in a car it might be the presence of a car close in front which causes problems. Some passengers have to travel in the back seat for this reason.

Drivers and passengers get symptoms driving under bridges or under high tension power cables. They may have to plan their route carefully so as to avoid these hazards. That may mean driving down a motorway and coming off at each interchange to avoid the motorway bridge.

Drivers can get their symptoms overtaking long vehicles on the motorway, or driving at speed, or having to sit at the front of a queue of traffic at traffic lights. Some of these situations can be quite disabling if you depend on your car. All of them are treatable, and the principles of treatment are the same as always.

You can begin by working out exactly what your problem is. You then practise it in your imagination, using relaxation exercises to help control your symptoms. Then it is time to get your car out and find a suitable place to practise the situations which you find difficult. Choose a safe quiet place and drive under the electricity cable, or the bridge, or whatever. It is more difficult to practise problems with overtaking or city driving, but it can be done. Choose a quiet time and quiet bit of road and find one truck to overtake. Take it steadily and evenly. You may feel tense, but you will be able to do it and when you have done it once you can do it again. You must do it again, over and over, until confidence returns.

Practise often and also learn to relax in your car.

Aircraft

Many people get their symptoms in aircraft. They are often not prepared to fly because of the symptoms they know they will experience in the aircraft. The problem of course is that once you are in an aircraft you can't very well get off. This is not an easy one to deal with because you can't fly every day. You can do relaxation exercises and you can imagine you are in a plane. You can look at pictures of a plane. You can, perhaps with the help of a tape recorder, go through the stages of flying from take-off to landing, in the quiet of your own room. You can anticipate your symptoms and learn to live with them.

In a way you are helped by the fact that once you are on a plane you can't get off it. You don't have that option. If you have the courage to get on then you will arrive. You must have the confidence to know that your symptoms will do you no harm. And you *can* practise the getting on bit. Go to the airport and watch the departures. Practise relaxing in the lounge. Watch the planes and relax while you are doing it. Relax at home and look at pictures of planes. Get used to the whole idea of planes.

When you get on the aircraft go through all the things you have practised at home. Put your head back. Breathe slowly and deeply. Slow everything down. Let your symptoms flow over you. Remember that they will peak at take-off and rapidly subside. Be prepared to ride out that peak. You might even enjoy your flight.

Landing is another difficult time in the flight. There is that awful moment when the plane seems to hang in space, and the ground seems a long way away. You can rehearse this in your mind, but it is difficult. Many ordinary people without anxiety states find this difficult. You have an advantage over them. You know how to relax, how to sit deeply in your chair and let the world go by. Your symptoms can do you no harm and you won't break down or make a fool of yourself. At worst you will be very very uncomfortable. Think of the joy of arriving.

Animals: dogs and cats

Some people who eventually find themselves confined to the house get into that situation because they develop severe symptoms when confronted by a dog or cat. This is a terrible tragedy because they can learn to deal with this situation if they go about it the right way.

Begin as always by practising relaxation exercises. When you are confident that you can relax adequately you should start to imagine that there is a dog close by you. If you have a good imagination you will experience some of the symptoms which you experience in the real situation and you can practise using relaxation to control them.

After a week or so doing this, you may be ready to consider going further. Don't progress until you feel ready. If you have difficulty using your imagination to conjure up the image of a dog or cat, use a picture of the animal. When you feel comfortable in your imagination you will have to introduce the animal itself. You will have to find a friend with a suitable dog or cat: a bouncy retriever would hardly be the best dog to use initially.

Your friend might bring the dog to your house, but if it is a cat or other animal you may have to go to the house where it lives. In either case, keep the animal out of sight, or at least keep it at a distance where it will not be threatening. Sit quietly and relax. As always, repeat the exercise until you are comfortable. Then progress at your own pace. Bring the animal nearer week by week until you can touch it. It may be a slow process, but this phobia can be disabling and it is worth taking time.

Your last step will be to go out and face animals in an uncontrolled environment. Take a friend. Don't avoid dogs but don't seek them out. Be prepared to walk past them. Later you will be able to pat dogs and stroke cats. It is not easy, but the rewards are tremendous.

Eating in restaurants

There are people who find that their gullet tightens when they tackle a meal. They may even have to leave the table in order to swallow. It is always worse when someone is watching, so it is inevitably worse in public, and eating in restaurants can be a problem. The situation can be difficult long before the food arrives. The smell of cooking produces salivation so that your stomach churns, and inevitably your body interprets this discomfort as panic. You may want to swallow. It may be warm, and there may be strange people with whom you have to converse. It can be very difficult.

Don't give in to panic. Assess the situation. What is happening? Are you sweating? Are you salivating? Are you just hungry?

When the meal arrives there can be the problem of muscle tension in the muscles of the gullet. It can be unpleasant, but you can make it less so if you try to relax, breathe deeply and eat slowly. Everyone else is eating so they won't be watching you.

If you have this problem you should practise managing it. That means eating in public as often as possible, which can be expensive these days. Choose a restaurant which you can go to often. Your local Chinese restaurant might be suitable. Choose a quiet time. Go with a friend and have one course. Eat slowly and relax. Go often and make the exercise more difficult. Go at a busier time. Sit in the middle where you can be seen. Take other friends. Slowly build up your experience and your confidence.

Small social gatherings

Meals with friends or small social get-togethers may be difficult. The method of approaching this is just the same as many already mentioned. Start in your imagination. Go to social events which seem to be less threatening than the one which causes your symptoms. When the time comes to go to a social gathering, choose some friends and admit to them that you are ill at ease in company. You might find it easier to invite them to your house in the first instance. You may feel safer on home ground. Use all your powers of relaxation. Keep the encounter short, perhaps just a few drinks. Talk quietly and pretend to be calm even if you don't feel it.

You can practise conversation in a mirror, or using a tape recorder. Meet the same people often and make the exercise more difficult by inviting strange people home or by going out to someone else's house.

Walking down a crowded street

This can be difficult for a number of reasons. We have already talked about animal phobias. Often it is just that you can't meet the eyes of the person walking towards you. You are uncertain how to react, or how they will react to you. You may be going out of your way to avoid busy streets.

Begin at home with a mirror. Practise looking at your own eyes so that you know what you look like to others. Practise smiling at people you know, and reacting to different people so that you know what you will look like if you have to pass them in the street.

Eventually you will have to go out and face real individuals. Start by taking walks down local streets with your husband or a friend. When you meet people glance at their eyes and glance away. Don't worry too much about what they think of you. That doesn't matter. Progress until you can walk down the main street of your own town, and keep practising.

Cinemas, theatre and church

This is another common problem. Some people get all sorts of symptoms in public places. They feel trapped in an auditorium. Quiet scenes, or the quiet movements in a concert performance, can produce feelings of panic or dizziness. Fortunately there are many cinemas and places of public entertainment around, so it isn't too difficult to find somewhere to practise.

The cinema is a good place to begin as it is less formal. You can come and go as you please so you feel less trapped. Go in the afternoon when it is quiet. Go with a friend. Take along some sweets which you can eat quietly. Choose a programme which really interests you so that you are not bored. Don't try an exciting, or worse, an erotic film or you will never relax. Watch out for the quiet bits which will make your symptoms worse. Sit near the door at the end of a row at first, though you must practise sitting in a more inaccessible place later on. Go often and make the practice more difficult by choosing a busy cinema or theatre at a busy time. As always be prepared for panic attacks. If you do get one, let it pass over you. Don't leave, it won't last more than a few seconds. Breathe deeply and slowly. You will find that your symptoms get less bothersome as time goes on.

Concern about the way you look

Some people feel that they look 'different' or that they project a bad image of themselves. They may feel that they are fat, or that they are repulsive because of some minor birth abnormality. Some people are embarrassed to undress in public for *no* reason, and there are people who avoid public places altogether because of concern about the way they look.

Begin by identifying the problem. Do you have a birth mark, or some physical abnormality? Are you too fat or too thin, and are these things important? Your fear may not be rational at all. You may have got things completely out of proportion.

If you are overweight you may want to lose weight, but this is very difficult. Surely it is better to accept the way you are, the way other people certainly accept you?

Begin with the mirror. You really aren't that bad. There a lot of people who look worse. In order to overcome your dislike of people looking at your body you will have to go somewhere where people can see you. The best place for this may be a public baths. Find one where you are unlikely to meet people you know. Go at a quiet time and don't stay too long. Take a friend. Get used to having your body on view.

You may be surprised to find that no one takes very much interest in you. If you do have a birth mark or some abnormality, don't try to hide it. It is better to learn to live with it. If children comment that is too bad. You will have to practise hearing that sort of comment until it doesn't matter any more. Once you really don't care, life can return to normal.

Being alone in the house

This can be difficult if you are a housewife and have to be alone part of the time. It may come about when all the children go to school. You may begin to get symptoms in the quiet house. Adolescent girls can also have this trouble, and it can come on after a burglary.

If you are alone you have plenty of time to practise your relaxation exercises. Always start when you are feeling comfortable. You can use them to control your symptoms later. When you begin to feel uncomfortable in the house by yourself, try to determine what is actually happening. What symptoms are you getting and what mechanism is bringing them on? It might be an upset stomach, or diarrohoea, or palpitations. Once you have identified the symptoms you will find them easier to control. Use your relaxation exercises. Don't ever be tempted to speed up and work harder and harder at the housework. Always slow down.

If things are so bad that you can't be by yourself in the house, arrange to be in the house with a friend or relative in another room. Extend the time you are in a room alone. Eventually you must try being in the house by yourself. Start by staying in the house for a few minutes and gradually build up the time, working to a programme.

Hand tremor in public

A hand tremor is always worse when someone is watching you. It can be embarrassing or worse if you work at a job such as being a cashier. Your tremor is caused by tense muscles so the trick in overcoming your tremor is again, relaxation. Sit at ease. Keep your hands in view but keep them relaxed. Again, start in the privacy of your own home. Pretend that people are watching you. Relax your shoulders. Move slowly and deliberately.

Do simple exercises at home. Try carrying a cup with a little water in it. At first it will rattle on the saucer. Try to control it. When you have made progress, fill the cup fuller. Keep at it until you can carry a full cup and saucer.

Carry this over into your work. Practise working slowly. Work out exercises you can practise. Gradually your tremor will get better.

Loud noise

Loud noise can be very bothersome to some individuals. That is no joke if you have teenage sons or daughters. It is easy to overcome if you go about it the right way. We all have televison sets and record players. Choose a time when you can be by yourself. Do your relaxation exercises in front of the television with the volume turned down low. Every day turn the volume up until you find a level that is uncomfortable. Keep it at that level until it becomes comfortable, which may take a few days. Then turn it up further. You should soon be able to stand quite loud noise.

After you have practised at home, you might try in other noisy places outside. A disco is intimidating for anyone. Eventually you should be able to manage a disco. Then you will know that you have beaten the problem.

Muscle pain

You may get severe cramping pain in the muscles of your legs or in your arms or chest. You must of course eliminate the possibility of physical disease by seeing your doctor. If there is no physical cause, set about tackling your problem. It is not an easy one to beat. The pain can be severe and frightening. You have to convince yourself that the pain can do you no harm. The source of your pain is muscle spasm, like a 'stitch' in the side.

Relaxing may help, but your pain is severe and it is not easy to relax. You really have to convince your body that the pain has no significance. To do this you have to confront your pain. Take it on. Instead of holding yourself tight, like someone in a cold wind, move around. Stretch the painful leg. If you were a runner you would have to 'run through' your cramp. That's what you have to do now. You have to exercise through your pain. Choose any exercise you like. Press-ups are useful for chest pain. Rapid walking or running may help leg pain. Once you *know* that your pain can do you no harm, it will gradually disappear.

Passing water in company

This is an exclusively male problem. Some men are unable to pass water in a public lavatory when there are other men present. There is no simple answer to this problem apart from the golden rule of finding a quiet place to start practising and practise often. If you persevere you will in time be able to use a public lavatory like anyone else.

Bed and sex

We all have the right to a happy fulfilled sex life. Sex should come naturally, but like many other things it can cause problems for some people. This is because the sexual act creates a situation which some people find threatening.

The treatment of such a problem is rather specialized, but the methods are based on the principles described in this book, and just as successful. Relaxation exercises can be used and one should start by reducing the situation to its least threatening form. The Marriage Guidance Council has some excellent books on the subject, or you might want to read another book in this series entitled *Successful Sex* by F.E. Kenyon. Your doctor may be able to refer you to someone who can help.

If you are to tackle your problem you need to understand what is actually going on, and to have an understanding partner. The first step therefore is to talk about your problem with your partner. See if you can work out what your difficulty actually is. Almost always there is a loss of confidence in your ability to manage the sexual act. It becomes very important that you perform adequately, and because it is important, tensions are produced which make normal intercourse difficult.

For women the problem tends to be a tightening of the muscles of the vagina. Muscle tightening is a common feature of many conditions mentioned in this book. As always, practise relaxation exercises, this time particularly in bed. Forget about intercourse for a while. There are other ways of showing affection. These need not lead on to intercourse until you are ready. What is it about intercourse which brings on this tightening? Often it is a feeling of being trapped, of having no control. It may be that the very position for the sexual act is threatening, making you feel trapped. Agree with your partner that you will not attempt intercourse until you are ready, and that it may take some time. Experiment a little and be prepared to take the initiative. Find a position which is not threatening and proceed from there. You and your partner must educate each other. It takes time and patience, but it can be done.

The two problems which tend to bother men are those of impotence, or failure to maintain an erection, and premature ejaculation. Men feel that a lot is expected of them in intercourse. A fear of failure makes intercourse threatening. Tension is produced and intercouse becomes difficult. The principles of treatment are the same. Learn to relax. Ban intercourse until you are ready for it. Show your affection in other ways. Explore your relationship and as confidence returns so will your capacity for sex.

Premature ejaculation is slightly different, but it is very treatable. Ban intercourse and concentrate on other things until you feel ready. Then you should practise control by beginning the sexual act but stopping short of ejaculation. You will need your partner's help and co-operation. It takes time as always, but it is worth it. The reward is a normal and happy sex life.

The underlying principle

There are almost as many causes of tension as there are people, and it is not possible to mention all of them. Some people for example, get symptoms in high winds or in thunder storms. Some people dread hospitals. Or it may be insects. It doesn't really matter so long as you understand what is actually happening to your body, and the principles which lie behind treatment.

You must learn to relax. You must reduce the problem to its least threatening form and practise it until you are confident. You must practise often and there must be no back-sliding. Work out a time-table and stick to it. Make your practice more difficult as confidence returns. Progress slowly.

It all takes time, but the rewards for time spent are tremendous.

6

Slow Down

There are many simple things which you can do which will help you on a day to day basis. There are little tricks which will help you to survive at parties or in shops. It is worth learning and practising them.

What do other people do?

Think about the actor or the televison personality. Before they go 'on the air' their pulse rate goes up alarmingly and they experience all sorts of symptoms which are produced by their nervous system. Yet they appear on the screen calm and relaxed. You would never know that they are uncomfortable or ill at ease, and yet nearly all of them are. They achieve this relaxed effect by practising relaxation and looking calm. They rehearse the things they are going to do and say. They are careful about their appearance and the way they look to other people. They look calm and relaxed, but all the time they have a lot of adrenalin pumping round their bodies.

You are just like that actor or television personality, except that your stress is not the stage or the television camera. Your stress is a situation in everyday life. You can learn from them.

At home

First of all think about the things you do at home when you are by yourself. Do you get symptoms at home when you are by yourself? You can usually tell when you are becoming physically tense, often in anticipation of some coming event. If you have practised your relaxation exercises it will be easier for you to spot when this is coming on. What do you do when this happens?

If you are like most people you will begin to speed up when there is a real need for you to slow down. The housewife will begin to clean the house furiously or rush to do the dishes, or perhaps to knit. The more vigorously she works the more adrenalin she produces, and the more tense she feels. She should sit down and slow down.

When you first feel the beginnings of tension you should start practising relaxation. Sit down for ten minutes and take it easy. You should try to find out what is making you tense. When you do go back to your housework you should work slowly and deliberately, perhaps listening to some quiet music while you do so. If there is a stressful situation in the offing, rehearse it in your mind. Most of all, slow down.

Anticipate

If you have a stressful event on the horizon, say a party or a dinner, spend some time by yourself relaxing, and when you are relaxed think about what will happen. Visualize the situation. Try to anticipate the event. Think what people will say and what you will say to them. If you have a vivid imagination you will experience the same feelings when you imagine the situations as you might feel if you were there.

Try to anticipate the problems which your anxiety state might give you. Anticipate the bad moments and how you might deal with them. I don't mean that you should find ways of avoiding them. You should decide how you will manage them so that they don't take you by surprise and make you panic.

You can copy the television personality in many ways. You will have a mirror and possibly a tape-recorder. It is very important for you to know that although you may *feel* strange, you certainly don't *look* strange, or sound strange. Even if your face is tense and tight, and talking seems to be a problem, you will always look and sound normal unless you do something silly like trying to hide behind sunglasses. You will have to learn to sit, talk, smile and walk normally despite the fact that you feel very strange and

41

your muscles feel tense enough to snap.

The next time you feel really bad, have a look at yourself in the mirror. Smile to yourself. Walk up and down. Look into your eyes. Practise a few words. Imagine you are on television and see what you look like. If you are nervous about talking, talk away to yourself. Pretend you are listening to someone else. Listening can be more difficult than talking. If you think you sound strained, tape yourself and you may be surprised how normal you sound.

Your appearance

Take care with your appearance. You are learning to act the part of normality. Like an actor, your dress helps you to feel the part. Conservative clothes and make-up will help.

When you are in company, remember that people don't observe you that closely. They are too busy trying to make an impression themselves. Sometimes they don't even listen to what you say. They are thinking about their own next pronouncement. Or they may have piles and be hoping that the itch will stop. Or their ulcer may be playing up. They get a sort of general impression of you and that is all, unless you want to make it otherwise.

So, if you are getting tense, the golden rule is to slow down. Talk slowly and quietly unstead of gabbling on. Move slowly. Gesture slowly. One of the most difficult things is to learn to manage silences, and you must do that. It is one of the things that an actor must practise. Don't jump in to fill a break in the conversation. Let someone else do that. You find something else to do. Look at your glass. Look at a picture on the wall or study your nails.

Panic

You should be prepared to manage panic. If you begin to feel tense and agitated, wonder why? Are you beginning to sweat? Is the dinner slow to come and is your stomach churning? Is the smell of food making you salivate? Are you trapped by a 'super-bore'? Is the music too loud?

Often there is a reason for the way you feel, and if you can find out the reason it is a great relief. An erotic or frightening episode in a film can put your pulse rate up and your body may interpret this as the beginning of panic. All sorts of other reactions may follow.

In the long run you may panic. It can happen to anyone. Panic attacks don't come out of the blue. With a little experience you can tell when they are coming on. If you know one is going to occur then it is less frightening. Don't leave the room or shop. A panic attack lasts seconds only. It will have gone almost as soon as you have closed the door. You will be outside with a feeling of defeat. Stay where you are. Let it flow over you. Wallow in the strange sensation. It isn't too unpleasant if you aren't frightened by it. It might help if you sit down or lean against a wall. You don't have to. You can continue a conversation despite having a panic attack. Every time you 'ride out' a panic attack you know that the next one will be easier. You will have won the battle and you will be on the way to winning the war. The same rules apply to panic attacks whenever you enounter them.

Communication

We communicate in many ways. We use our eyes and our gestures. Eye to eye contact is an important part of our communication with others, and it is something which some people find difficult. If you look into someone's eyes too much you may seem aggressive or cause them embarrassment: too little and you may seem disinterested. Practise talking to yourself in the mirror. Practise talking to friends. Correct use of eye to eye contact may be something you will have to learn.

Don't draw attention to yourself

Practise sitting in a relaxed way, with your hands resting on the arms of your chair or on your lap. Don't over-do gestures. They should come naturally as part of your conversation. Make your gestures slow and deliberate.

Never draw attention to yourself by the things you say unless you really want to. The person who is ill at ease may feel that he has to make excuses for himself. He may complain about the heat. He may enter a room announcing at the same time that he cannot stay. There is absolutely no need to make excuses for the way you feel you might appear. Your appearance is almost certainly entirely normal and no one will have noticed that you are ill at ease. The person who is quiet and says little is usually considered to be wise.

All this sounds very simple, and for some people it is. Usually these 'social skills' do not need to be learned. You may not be so lucky. You may have been learning the wrong lessons for years. It is time you started to learn the right ones.

You must know that however agitated or ill at ease you may *feel*, you will look and sound comfortable and relaxed. When you are confident that this is the case, life will be much easier.

7

Your Future

No matter how severe your symptoms are they can be improved. No matter how many situations you may find difficult to face, you can be helped. It doesn't matter how long you have had your problem. Occasionally you may hear of someone who has been housebound for forty years. With a little help she has been able to overcome her symptoms and go out. It is a tragedy that she was not helped forty years earlier.

What can you expect?

It is quite possible that your symptoms may be cured completely. Certainly they can be made manageable, and that is what you really want. You want to be the one who manages your symptoms rather than have your symptoms manage you. You want the pleasure factor replaced in your life. You want to enjoy your social contacts again. You want to enjoy going out again, and that *can* be achieved. You can lead a full and happy life.

You must begin to seek out and tackle your problems from every angle you can. Seek help wherever you can find it. You might be surprised how helpful your doctor can be, particularly if you don't insist that you have a physical condition and demand a physical cure. If you and he can agree about your anxiety state he may be able to give you help or advice or even put you in touch with someone who is an expert in the field. At the end of the day however, *you* must do the work if you want to overcome your condition. There just is no easy way.

Your doctor may offer you medication. This is likely to be a tranquillizer such as valium. These drugs have the effect of relaxing muscles and can be extremely useful in the short term. They may help you to get started on the road to recovery, but do not come to depend on them. Use them in the short term if your doctor agrees. You might like to use them just before a stressful event. They may help you to find your feet at a party or getting on a train, bus or plane. These are things for you to discuss with your doctor. Do not rely too much on drugs. Rely on yourself. That is the only way.

There are tablets which will help you in other ways. There are tablets which will help to regulate your heart rate for example. If palpitations or a racing heart are your problems, these tablets will help you. Other tablets help control diarrhoea. If this is a problem in difficult situations, they may help you face them. Use them carefully as your doctor prescribes them, and do not come to depend on them.

Do not use alcohol to control your symptoms

Alcohol is a drug and an addictive one at that. Many alcoholics have anxiety states and begin their alcoholism because they find that initially alcohol makes their symptoms easier to manage. A few drinks at a party can do no harm. Drinks before you go out should be avoided. If you have to drink before you go out in the morning then you already are an alcoholic. Rely on yourself, not on alcohol. With this condition, you ultimately have to come to have confidence in yourself and to depend on your own resources. There is no easy way.

Other cures

Some people will try anything to overcome their symptoms, often at great expense. There will be many advertisements in both local and national papers for patent cures. Try to avoid quacks. If there is one in your area the chances are that your doctor will know about them.

Hypnotism may be useful if practised by an expert and if you are a susceptible subject. It is uneven in the results it achieves. There is nothing magical about it. It is really just a form of very deep relaxation. If you go to a hypnotist, make sure he is competent and qualified. Some doctors and clinical psychologists practise hypnosis, and your doctor may be able to put you in touch with someone suitable. There are other cures advertised. Acupuncture is currently in vogue. Again, seek an expert, and not someone who has bought a book of instructions and a set of needles. Homeopathy, naturopathy, chiropractic and the like don't seem to have a lot to offer.

Help will come from something which you do for yourself, not from something someone does to you. Yoga teaches relaxation and self control. It can be useful and has the advantage of involving you with other people. You should begin to get together with groups of people. If there is a self-help group, or some form of group therapy in your area, give it a try.

Here are a few addresses:

The Phobics Society
4 Cheltenham Road
Chorlton-cum-Hardy
Manchester M21 1QN

The Phobic Trust
25A The Grove
Coulsdon
Surrey CR2 2BH

The Open Door Association
447 Pensby Road
Heswall
Wirral
Merseyside L61 9PQ

Stresswatch
9 Poland Street
London

Your lifestyle

You should look at your lifestyle and see if there are any ways in which you could change it and begin to mix with other people in a sympathetic environment. I don't mean that you should suddenly develop interests that you didn't have before. Don't run out and buy an expensive camera just so that you can join the local photographic club. See what things interest you. You might go along to the historical society. You might want to go somewhere where you are not known at first. Do go to places where you can get to know people, and where you will have mutual interest. Find things that your spouse can share with you.

Don't be afraid to discuss your problem with others, but be careful who you discuss it with. You can lose an acquaintance very quickly if you start to unload your problems on to him. People don't know how to react to someone with an anxiety state if they have no knowledge what it means to suffer from one. If you are with someone you know well there is no harm in saying that you tend to be uneasy in company, or on trains, or whatever. Don't make a big thing out of it. If he or she understands then you will know by their responses. People close to you can be of most help. Involve them in your treatment. Let them read this book. You can rely on people you love and trust.

You have the whole of your life in front of you. You want it to be pleasant and relaxed. You want it to be enjoyable: to enjoy the things that other people take for granted. There is no reason why you should not be able to do this. You can overcome your difficulties. Many people have done so before.

Begin today. Plan your attack carefully, using the tables and charts in Part Two of this book. You must have strict discipline and there must be no backsliding. Your world will improve rapidly. You will have set-backs and bad days. Expect them. Look at your overall progress. It will be slow but very sure. Whatever your problem, it can be overcome if you have the right approach and the right attitude.

Don't be too serious about your exercises. A sense of humour will help in the end in all your adventures.

So get started right away, and good luck!

PART TWO

1

The General Questionnaire

Please do not read this section until you have read and fully understood Part One. When you are sure that you understand the principles which lie behind this method of dealing with your problems, you can start doing the exercises outlined here. It will take you several weeks to get through the course so don't be in a hurry. Proceed one step at a time.

The object of this questionnaire is to get you to know a little more about yourself. Don't take it too seriously and don't attempt to be too introspective. You shouldn't try to find the cause of your problems in your past. Concentrate on the future. You must see yourself as you really are. You must have no illusions about yourself. You must certainly not underestimate yourself.

You cannot change your character or your nature. I'm sure you don't want to do that anyway. What you do want to do is to be yourself, to fulfil your potential and never to have to say, 'I could be such-and-such if only I did not have this anxiety state.'

The target which you are going to set yourself must be something which you can achieve. If you are honest about this, then you will have no difficulty in overcoming your problems.

Now do the questionnaire. There are numbers in the 'Yes/No' columns. Put a ring around the number in the appropriate 'yes' or 'no' box. At the end of each section add up your score. The scoring is arbitrary and is meant as a guide only. The total score obtainable and an acceptable average score will be given after the questionnaire.

If you score highly, then your problem will be more difficult to deal with. If you have a very low score, then there may be less difficulty. No matter how high your score may be, you can be helped.

Now do the questionnaire; the comments follow on.

50

THE GENERAL QUESTIONNAIRE

Put a ring round your score
in the appropriate column.

SECTION 1

	Yes	No
Did you have a happy childhood?	0	1
Did your parents live together?	0	1
Did you have any brothers and sisters?	0	1
Did you get on well with them?	0	1
Were you a 'bed wetter'?	2	0
Were you a nail biter?	1	0
Were you a shy child?	1	0
Did you belong to youth organizations?	0	1
Were you happy in them?	0	1
Were your parents strict?	1	0

Score

SECTION 2

	Yes	No
Did you enjoy school?	0	1
Were you a popular child?	0	1
Were you academically bright?	0	1
Were you good at games?	0	1
Were you bullied?	2	0
Had you many hobbies?	0	1
Did you have many friends?	0	2

Score

SECTION 3

	Yes	No
As an adolescent, did you have any girlfriends/boyfriends?	0	1
Were you attracted to members of the opposite sex?	0	1
Did you get on well with your parents?	0	1
Did your parents understand you?	0	2
Did you indulge in sport?	0	1
Did you have any serious hobbies?	0	1
Did you go on to college?	0	1
Would you have liked to go on to further education?	1	0
Are you happy in your choice of occupation?	0	2
Is your job too demanding?	1	0

Score:

SECTION 4

	Yes	No
Are you an ambitious person?	0	2
Are you an outgoing person?	0	2
Do people like you?	0	2
Are you a sensitive person?	0	1
Do you cry easily?	1	0
Do you get depressed?	1	0
Have you ever considered suicide?	2	0
Are you a lonely person?	2	0
Do you find life boring?	1	0
Do you wish you had more interesting things to do?	0	1
Have you many friends?	0	1
Are you married?	0	2
Are you happy with your spouse?	0	2
Does your spouse understand your problem?	0	2
Do you go out with your spouse at least once a week?	0	1

Score

SECTION 5

	Yes	No
Have you always been tense and anxious?	3	0
Have you recently become tense?	0	1
Have you had a recent change in you personal circumstances?	0	2
Have you recently had a child?	0	1
Have you had any frightening or unpleasant experiences?	0	2

Score

SECTION 6

Are you a reasonably attractive person?	0	1
Are you shy in company?	1	0
Do you have difficulty meeting peoples' eyes?	1	0
Do you feel awkward walking down a crowded street?	1	0
Do you feel awkward in company?	2	0
Do you ever leave a place because you feel tense?	2	0
Do you smoke a lot?	1	0
Do you talk too much in company?	1	0
Do important people frighten you?	1	0
Do people like you?	0	2

Score

SECTION 7

	Yes	No
Are you prepared to put time into the problem of overcoming your anxiety state?	0	4
Do you avoid difficult situations?	3	0
Are you symptoms frightening?	2	0
Do you believe that this book can help you?	0	3
Are you prepared to put a major effort in to overcoming your tension state?	0	4
If you weren't tense, would you be satisfied with the sort of person you are?	0	3
	Score	

Exercise

Write a few paragraphs about yourself based on your answers. What sort of a person are you? How did your childhood affect you? Write an honest appraisal of yourself both now and as you were growing up. Imagine that you are talking to a therapist.

. Now look to the future. If the restrictions placed upon you by your anxiety state are removed, what sort of person is left? What way will your life be changed? You should have portrait of the person and the life-style you are seeking to achieve. Is that worth working for?

2

Explanation of the Questionnaire

Section 1

If you had an unhappy childhood or come from a broken home you are more likely to have problems in adulthood. If you were a shy child and perhaps a nail biter or a bed wetter, then perhaps you have always been an anxious person. You may have begun to avoid difficult situations and learn the wrong lessons as a very young child. That doesn't mean that you will necessarily have more difficulty overcoming your problems. You may have been an aggressively normal child and still become a tense adult. You can't change what is past and you can't blame anyone. Your childhood experience is part of your personality now. You should deal with the present and forget the past.

Maximum score: 11. Most people should score below 6.

Section 2

It is at school that we first learn to interact with people outside our immediate family. Some of us do it well by instinct. Some of us are more reticent and find it difficult. Some do not succeed at all. If your difficulties were apparent at school then it may be more difficult for you to unlearn the old wrongly-learned lessons. It is not impossible. If your personality before the onset of your anxiety state was entirely normal, then you may quickly get over your problems.

Maximum score: 9. Most people should score below 5.

Section 3

As an adolescent you begin to react with members of the opposite sex. It can be a time of great difficulty. It can also be a time when you begin to find ways of dealing with your problems. If you made the wrong decisions then you may be paying the price for them now. You may have withdrawn into yourself. Some of the factors involved in keeping your anxiety state going may have started then. You may have taken on a job which is too demanding, or perhaps not demanding enough.

Maximum score: 12. Most people should score below 7.

Section 4

What are you really like now? There may be more to your problems than simple anxiety. Perhaps you have difficulties over excessive loneliness. If you are depressed then you should see your doctor. He will be able to help you. If you have problems with your marriage then you should try to sort them out. Seek professional help. The Marriage Guidance Council offers an excellent service. Is drink a problem? Alcoholics Anonymous can be useful. Perhaps you should change your life-style in small ways.

Maximum score: 23.   Most people score below 13.

Section 5

What triggered off your anxiety state? If it started suddenly, or as a result of a stressful situation which has now gone, it should get better quickly if you take it in hand. If it has been with you for years, then it will take more work and more time. It will get better if you are prepared to do the work.

Maximum score: 9.   Most people score below 5.

Section 6

You must spend time working on the things which you are doing wrong. If you have read Part One of this book then you will know what you should be doing about these things.

Maximum score: 13.   Most people score below 10.

Section 7

What are you prepared to do about your anxiety state? Is your attitude to it right? Have you enough motivation? All these things are very important. You must really want to get better. That is half the battle.

Maximum score: 19.   Most people score below 5.

3

Relaxation Exercises

Before you start to do anything else in the way of overcoming your symptoms you must take a week, or as long as is necessary to learn to relax. It is a very important skill to master and it is essential if you are to be successful in overcoming your problems.

Start practising it by yourself and then try it in other situations.

Read the passage about relaxation before you try anything. Don't try to tackle threatening situations until you have confidence in your ability to relax.

Enjoy your relaxation. It is a pleasant sensation.

What is relaxation?

Relaxation is a physical skill which can help you to overcome physical and mental tension. The exercises described later will teach you to relax, firstly by concentrating on noticing where your muscles tense and relax. Then as you practise and become more aware of the state of your muscles you will be able to control them and relax more deeply and more quickly. This is useful in helping you to relax at home, and also when you have acquired the skill, it will be useful to you in stressful situations outside. Learning what it feels like to be relaxed will help you to recognize when you are becoming tense, so that you can relax before you feel really bad. Do not expect to relax or to concentrate fully while you are a beginner. Expect to produce gradual progress day by day.

Preparing for relaxation exercises

Choose a quiet time and place to practise. Allow 20−30 minutes. Begin by lying on your back or sitting comfortably in an

59

armchair. Do not cross your arms or legs. Breathe slowly and deeply. Concentrate on the breathing movements in your chest, back and stomach. You may prefer to close your eyes or to look at a particular object or place. Breathe slowly and deeply.

Relaxing hands and arms

Try to keep the rest of your body relaxed and then clench your right fist. Notice the feelings of tension in your fingers, your thumb, the palm of your hand, your knuckles and the back of your hand. Keep your fist clenched and notice the feelings of tension in your wrist and lower part of your arm. Notice how clenching your fist makes your arm tense as well. Now, still concentrating, let your hand suddenly relax. Let your fingers hang and notice how they feel *warm* when you relax them. Notice also how your arm feels *heavy*. These feelings of heaviness and warmth are an important sign that you are succeeding in relaxing. Breathe slowly and concentrate on your right hand for a few more seconds. Next switch your attention to your left hand. Go through the same procedure as with your right hand. Clench your fist, concentrating to pinpoint all the different muscles which tense as you do this. Relax your left hand suddenly, and again try to notice feelings of heaviness and warmth. Let your breathing become slow and regular after each tension exercise. Both arms feel heavy.

Relaxing shoulder, neck and face

Now concentrate on the area around your shoulders and the upper parts of your arms, chest and back. Tense the muscles here by hunching up your shoulders. Hold them in that uncomfortable position and notice the muscle tension across the top of your shoulders, in your neck, in the top part of your chest and back, and in your arms. Notice your breathing is affected by tensing these muscles. Then, quite suddenly let these muscles relax. Let your arms become soft and heavy again and let your shoulders slump as low as possible. Your breathing becomes slow and regular again and you feel much more comfortable. Your arms are still and heavy and your shoulders are sagging as low as possible.

Concentrate next on your neck muscles. Tense them by pushing your head back. Be careful not to tense too hard. Push your head back only slightly. Notice the feelings of tension in the back of your neck, back of your head and across your shoulders. Notice the tension in the front of your neck and around your jaw and the lower part of your face. Now bring your head forward and suddenly let your neck muscles relax. Your head drops forward and feels floppy and heavy. Your breathing becomes slower and regular.

The next group of muscles are those in your face. Begin by frowning and creasing your forehead. Now add to the tension by closing your eyes as tightly as you can. Notice the feelings of tension you are producing. Make your face still more tense by clenching your jaws, pursing your lips and pressing your tongue against the roof of your mouth. Feel the tension in your cheeks and all around your face. Suddenly relax your face muscles. Notice the skin becoming soft as your forehead and cheeks return to normal and your jaw sags. Your mouth may be slightly open. Your breathing once again returns to normal. Now your arms and your head feel heavy, your shoulders are slumped, and your face feels soft. Breathe slowly.

Relaxing back and stomach muscles

Concentrate on the feelings in your back and produce tension by arching your back slightly. Hold the tension and try to notice where the muscles in your back are working. Suddenly let your back become soft and relaxed. Enjoy the contrast. Your breathing slows.

Next, tense your stomach muscles by pulling your stomach in so that you look as thin as possible. Hold it and concentrate on the tension. Gently let your stomach return to normal and notice how comfortable you feel when the muscles across your stomach are soft and relaxed. Breathe slowly and regularly.

Relaxing feet and legs

Concentrate on your right foot and right leg. Straighten your leg (but if you are sitting in a chair keep your heel on the floor). Now point your toes down away from you. Curl your toes under. Feel the tension in your toes, the sole of the foot, the upper part of the foot and the ankle. Notice the tension in the lower part of your leg, in the calf muscles and behind your knee. Feel it in the front of your knee and in the thigh muscles, right up to the top of the leg. Suddenly let your foot and leg relax. Your foot feels soft and floppy and your leg feels heavy and lazy. Again your breathing slows.

Now repeat this procedure with your left leg. Remember to concentrate as you tense and relax.

Finishing a relaxation session

Your breathing is now very slow and gentle. Your arms, legs and head are heavy, your face, neck and shoulders and stomach are soft. Enjoy the changes you have produced. Now think 'Calm' each time you breathe out. Repeat this 10−20 times.

Finish the session gradually. Let your muscles get ready to move again as you think 'Three-two-one-awake'.

How to use relaxation

1 Practise every day. Until you are skilled you should choose a time to practise when you are feeling fairly calm. With more practice you will be able to relax when you feel tense.

2 You may find that a tape recording of yourself or somebody else speaking the relaxation exercises is helpful.

3 Remember to use parts of the relaxation exercises to calm yourself when you meet problems in everyday life. Breathe

slowly and deeply, and let your arms be still and heavy when you feel tension building up. You can do this even in crowded places.

4   Many people find relaxation can help them get to sleep.

4

Symptom Questionnaire

This questionnaire is designed to find out exactly what symptoms you are experiencing. At the moment it is only a mass of amorphous sensations—a feeling of panic, or of severe discomfort. It is very difficult to improve vague symptoms. Your problem must be reduced to a list of definite symptoms. We can tackle symptoms where we cannot tackle just a feeling of unwellness.

The questionnaire is a list of symptoms. Tick the ones which you experience worst. You might find it easier if you carry the list with you and tick off symptoms at the time they happen.

SYMPTOM QUESTIONNAIRE

	Yes	No
Do you ever feel a wave of panic which seems to come from your feet and quickly spreads over your entire body? You feel dizzy and sweat and have a strong urge to leave the room?		
Do you ever experience muscle tension in your neck and shoulders?		
Do you get severe headaches that begin in the neck and spread across the scalp to affect the face and eyes? They may last several days.		
Do you ever get severe pain in the chest, arms or legs?		
Does your hand shake when people are watching you?		
Do you ever feel excessively tired during the day?		
Do you get diarrhoea in the mornings or before an important event?		
Do you get frequent loose stools?		
Do you get bouts of dizziness for no obvious reason?		
Do you get a feeling of severe tension around the eyes or grittiness in the eyes so that you feel that you are about to cry?		
Do you feel your stomach to be distended and uncomfortable?		
Do you feel your heart beating quickly or missing a beat?		
Do you sometimes feel that you can't get a full breath?		
Do you sometimes feel that you can't swallow, particularly in public?		
Do you ever have difficulty with sexual intercourse?		

If you have other symptoms write them in below:

65

5

Situation Questionnaire

People with anxiety states are often vague about their symptoms and also about the situations which make them worse. It is very difficult to deal with vague ideas. Much of this book is given over to persuading you to be precise about the things that cause you problems.

Some people deny completely that any situations cause them problems, when it is obvious that some situations can be very stressful. Fill in the questionnaire as honestly as you can. You may have to write in your own stressful situation. I have just suggested a few of the more common ones.

You might like to read the next page before proceeding, particularly if you have difficulty pinpointing difficult situations. You could fill in this questionnaire after you have kept a diary for a week.

If you have problems with tension which interfere with your sex life you should consult one of the many books on the subject. The Marriage Guidance Council could advise you. Their address is in the telephone book. The techniques for dealing with this type of problem are similar to the techniques outlined in this book.

SITUATION QUESTIONNAIRE

	Yes	No
Are you uncomfortable in the presence of other people?		
Are you uncomfortable in small rooms?		
Are you uncomfortable at home watching television?		
Do you have difficulty meeting peoples' eyes?		
Do you get symptoms in crowded rooms?		
Do you have trouble walking down the street?		
Do you get symptoms at work?		
Are your symptoms worse when people are watching you?		
Do you have difficulty talking on the telephone?		
Do you have symptoms on buses or trains?		
Do you have symptoms driving your car?		
Do you have symptoms as a passenger?		
Can you travel on motorways?		
Can you go under bridges?		
Do you have trouble on trains?		
Do you have symptoms in a lift?		
Do you have symptoms in an aircraft?		
Do you have symptoms when confronted by a dog or cat?		
Do you get your symptoms when birds are present?		
Do you have trouble eating in a restaurant?		
Do you get your symptoms in the church or cinema?		
Do you get your symptoms in shops?		
Do you get your symptoms in bed during intercourse?		
Do you avoid any situations which you know will bring on your symptoms?		

6

Situation Diary: How to Use it

No matter how well you think you understand your symptoms and the things which make them worse, it is worth your while keeping a diary for a week or so. Even if you are quite sure that your symptoms are always the same, keep the diary. You might be surprised how your symptoms fluctuate during a week and there might be clues as to what situations are making them worse. It is easier to organize your treatment if you have got this variation in your symptoms.

Keep the diary in some detail. Make a note of your main symptoms at the top. Then note below when they get worse. Note what might be making them worse. It may not just be a difficult situation like a bus journey. It might be an encounter with someone whom you find intimidating. It might even be the thought of something you are going to have to do.

Record how severe your symptoms are by writing a number from 1-5 in the space. Write 1 if the symptoms are mild and 5 if they are very severe. At the end of the week have a look at your diary and see what situations, or what particular aspects of a situation have caused you most bother. You could make a note of them at the bottom.

What symptoms give you most trouble? (Refer to your Symptom Questionnaire and write in your worst symptom/symptoms here.)

Record severity of symptoms in box (1-5).
Make a note of situation you are in at the time.

Days of the week. (Start recording on any day.)	MORNING	AFTERNOON	EVENING
MONDAY	(1-5) Severity: situation:	Severity: situation:	Severity: situation:
TUESDAY	Severity: situation:	Severity: situation:	Severity situation:
WEDNESDAY	Severity: situation:	Severity: situation:	Severity: situation:
THURSDAY	Severity: situation:	Severity: situation:	Severity situation:
FRIDAY	Severity: situation:	Severity: situation:	Severity: situation:
SATURDAY	Severity: situation:	Severity: situation:	Severity: situation:
SUNDAY	Severity: Situation:	Severity: Situation:	Severity: Situation:

What situations make your symptoms worse?

What situations do you avoid?

7

Plan of Campaign

You have now collected a lot of information and should have a good understanding of your problem and the factors which keep it going. Now is the time to plan your treatment of it. You may have found that reading the explanations and doing the relaxation exercises will have helped. There is much more that you can do.

Sit down with a pencil and paper and plan your compaign. You probably find the world a little hostile, and you will need help if you are to face it. A good plan of campaign, which you work out in advance and stick to, will be of great assistance. So will encouragement from your family and friends.

You will by now know what situations you find difficult. You cannot be expected to face your most difficult situation right away. You must 'creep up' on it by starting to practise your least threatening situation. You should only pass on to your next most threatening when you have mastered the one before. Avoid testing yourself. Stick to the programme. Expect bad days. If things are bad for a day or two go back to an easier stage and continue from there. You will never have to go back to the beginning.

Avoid back-sliding. The greatest danger is that you will not have the patience to persevere. It is easy to make excuses for yourself. This is where the diary forms will help.

It may take some thought and ingenuity to think of a list of situations which you can practise regularly and which will be of suitable difficulty. Do the best you can.

What is the most difficult situation you might have to face in your every-day life? This is the target you are aiming at. You wish to be comfortable in this situation.

Write it down ....

Think of a situation which is only slightly difficult. It brings on your symptoms only a little. It must be something you can practise every day.

1   Write it down ....

Now write down a situation which is only slightly more threatening and which you can practise every day.

2   Write it down ....

Think of your next most difficult situation.

3   Write it down ....

Now your next most difficult situation.

4   Write it down ....

Now go to the target situation which you noted at the top of the page. If you think you have made a list of enough situations in between, write your final target situation in now and you have completed your plan of campaign.

5   Target situation ....

Make a start by practising your first situation. Do it every day using all the advice in the book to help you. As soon as you have started to tackle your problem you will feel better.

8

Target Forms

Your greatest problem is keeping at it. You will always be tempted to 'back-slide'. A pencil and paper is of great value. You can look back over your programme and see whether you have been keeping honestly to the tasks you have set yourself. Keep these diary forms carefully. Make out one for each stage of your programme. Write your target in at the top and make a note of what you did and how you think you coped. Only when you have satisfied yourself that you have mastered the situation can you proceed.

Make out your own target forms for each stage of your progress. Write down the task you have set yourself in the appropriate place for each day.

Continue to record the severity of your symptoms (1-5) as before on the same forms and make a note of any unusual events, such as a panic attack or a particular success that you have.

Take note of any areas which will require further practice.

Progress will be slow, and you may find this disappointing. Keep your target forms and go back over them from time to time. It will help you to measure progress. Count the number of times you had bad symptoms. You will find that you have been making more progress than you thought.

TARGET FORMS   Make out your own

TARGET:

DAY	MORNING	AFTERNOON	EVENING
MONDAY			
TUESDAY			
WEDNESDAY			
THURSDAY			
FRIDAY			
SATURDAY			
SUNDAY			

9

Recording Progress

It is useful to see how you are getting on. Progress is slow, and it is not always easy to see improvement. Some sort of visual recording is helpful, and so a graph has been included. If you are keeping target forms you will have figures week by week. There is a maximum of five points for each morning, afternoon and evening. 'Five' is the maximum score, the most severe your symptoms can be. 'One' is the least severe.

The maximum score for a week is 105. Not many people will have this sort of score.

Carry the target forms with you and fill them in at the time. You can never remember symptoms afterwards. At the end of a week add up your score and mark it off on the graph opposite. The scale is entirely arbitrary. You can keep the graph longer by making out your own target forms.

Even if you don't keep detailed records for five or six weeks, it is useful to keep a record of a week towards the end of your treatment course so that you can compare it with previous records.

RECORDING PROGRESS

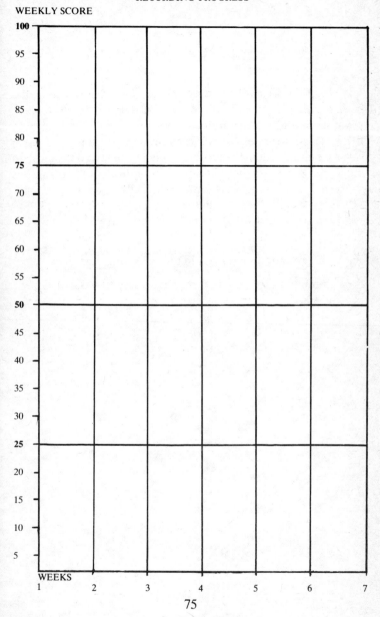

WEEKLY SCORE

100
95
90
85
80
75
70
65
60
55
50
45
40
35
30
25
20
15
10
5

WEEKS
1   2   3   4   5   6   7

75

10

Final Questionnaire

You should be well on the way to sorting out your problem. Have a look at Part One of the book now and again. There is a lot of advice in it and it helps to have a look at it from time to time. Progress will continue for some time. Keep working at it. Keep thinking up new ideas which might help. Never avoid the difficult situation. Keep relaxing. Keep practising. Keep rehearsing.

There is one last questionnaire. It is really just to round things off. Keep it until you feel that you have finished your course of self-treatment. It will help you to assess yourself. See how you do.

Put a ring round the numbers in the appropriate column.

A maximum score is 22. You should be able to score about 16.

FINAL QUESTIONNAIRE

	Yes	No
Did you carry out the instructions in the book carefully?	1	0
Did you practise the relaxation exercises?	1	0
Did you succeed in achieving deep relaxation?	2	0
Did you stop avoiding difficult situations?	3	0
Did you keep the target forms as suggested?	1	0
Do you still practice relaxation occasionally?	1	0
Can you relax in difficult situations?	2	0
Are you symptoms less frightening than they were before?	1	0
Are your symptoms less severe?	2	0
Do you still experience symptoms?	1	0
Can you now do things you couldn't do before?	1	0
If you ever had problems again could you think of ways of helping yourself?	2	0
Are you more confident than you were before?	1	0
Has this book helped you?	2	0
Could you help others?	1	0

Score:

Keep working!   Keep relaxing!   Good luck!

Index

Overcoming Common Problems Series

Overcoming Common Problems Series

How to Cope with your Nerves
DR TONY LAKE

How to Cope with Tinnitus and Hearing Loss
DR ROBERT YOUNGSON

How to do What You Want to Do
DR PAUL HAUCK

How to Enjoy Your Old Age
DR B. F. SKINNER AND M. E.
VAUGHAN

How to Interview and Be Interviewed
MICHELE BROWN AND
GYLES BRANDRETH

How to Love and be Loved
DR PAUL HAUCK

How to Say No to Alcohol
KEITH McNEILL

How to Sleep Better
DR PETER TYRER

How to Stand up for Yourself
DR PAUL HAUCK

How to Start a Conversation and Make Friends
DON GABOR

How to Stop Smoking
GEORGE TARGET

Jealousy
DR PAUL HAUCK

Learning to Live with Multiple Sclerosis
DR ROBERT POVEY, ROBIN DOWIE
AND GILLIAN PRETT

Living with Grief
DR TONY LAKE

Living with High Blood Pressure
DR TOM SMITH

Loneliness
DR TONY LAKE

Making Marriage Work
DR PAUL HAUCK

Making the Most of Middle Age
DR BRICE PITT

Making the Most of Yourself
GILL COX AND SHEILA DAINOW

Making Relationships Work
CHRISTINE SANDFORD AND WYN
BEARDSLEY

Meeting People is Fun
How to overcome shyness
DR PHYLLIS SHAW

No More Headaches
LILIAN ROWEN

One Parent Families
DIANA DAVENPORT

Overcoming Tension
DR KENNETH HAMBLY

The Parkinson's Disease Handbook
DR RICHARD GODWIN-AUSTEN

Second Wife, Second Best?
Managing your marriage as a second wife
GLYNNIS WALKER

Self-Help for your Arthritis
EDNA PEMBLE

The Sex Atlas
DR ERWIN HAEBERLE

Six Weeks to a Healthy Back
ALEXANDER MELLEBY

Solving your Personal Problems
PETER HONEY

A Step-Parent's Handbook
KATE RAPHAEL

Stress and your Stomach
DR VERNON COLEMAN

Overcoming Common Problems Series